THE PICTURE BOOK OF

NATURAL WONDERS

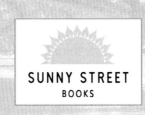

SUNNY STREET
BOOKS

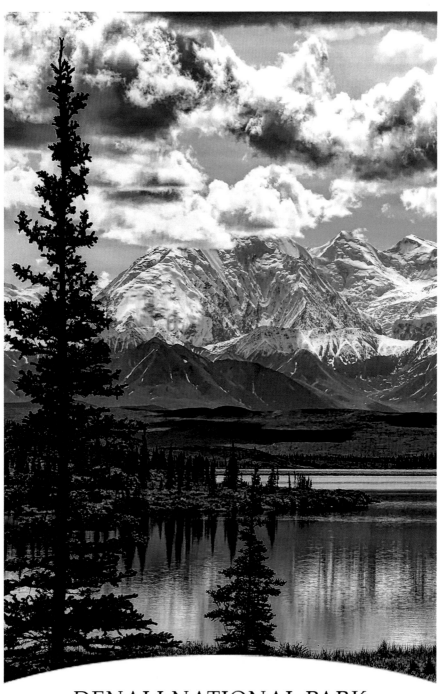

DENALI NATIONAL PARK
Alaska, United States

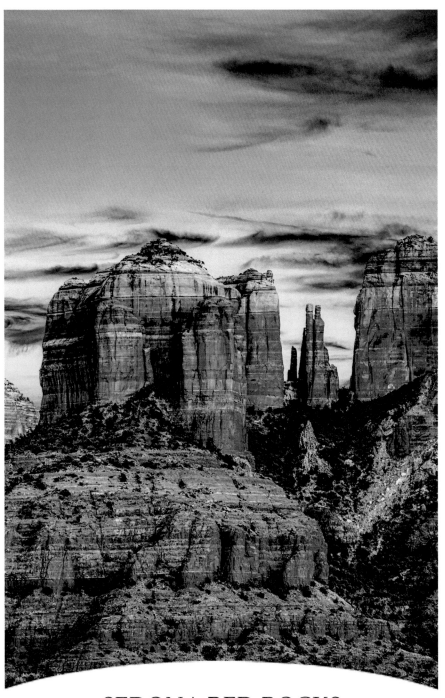

SEDONA RED ROCKS
Arizona, United States

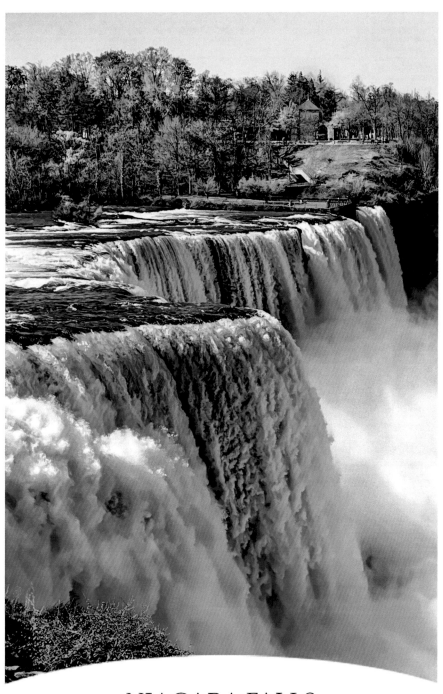

NIAGARA FALLS
Border of New York and Ontario

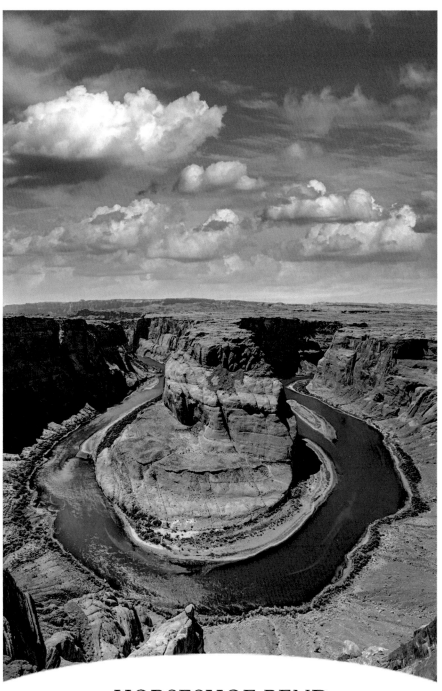

HORSESHOE BEND
Arizona, United States

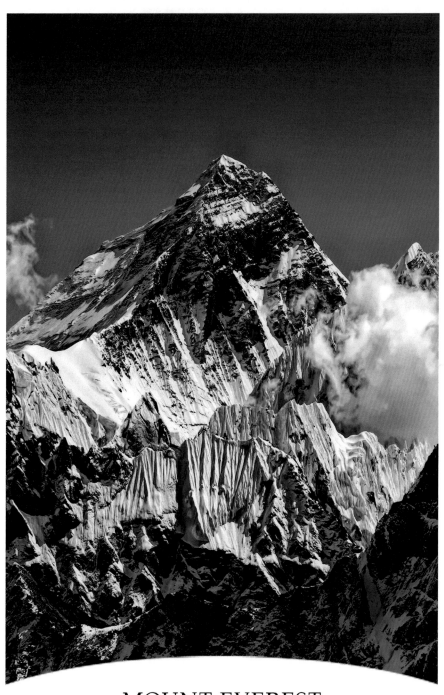

MOUNT EVEREST
Nepal/China Border

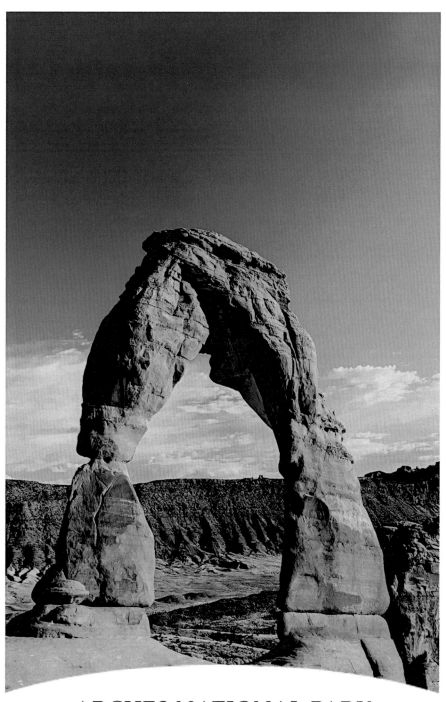

ARCHES NATIONAL PARK
Utah, United States

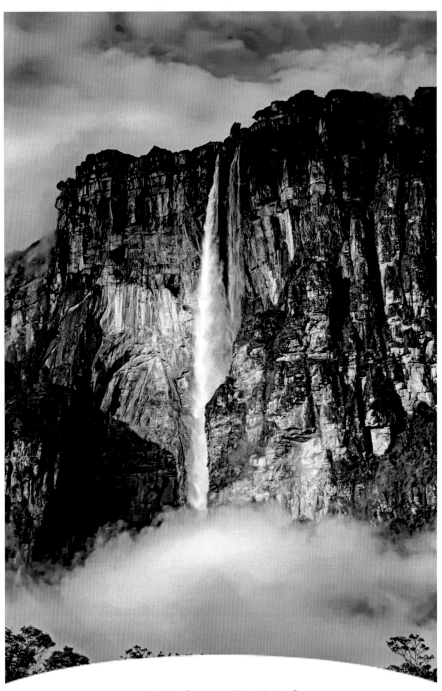

ANGEL FALLS
Canaima National Park, Venezuela

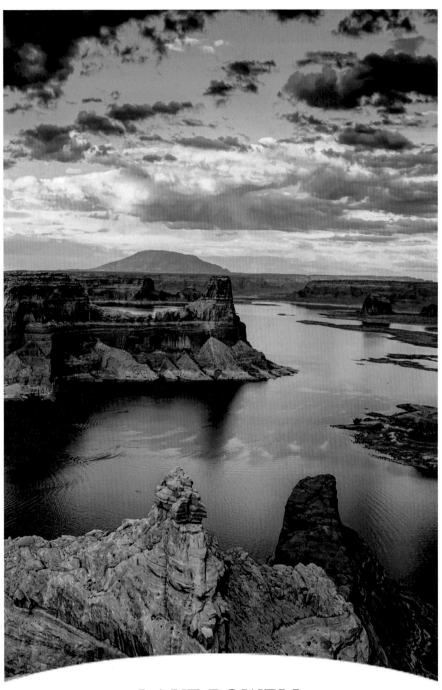

LAKE POWELL
Utah and Arizona, United States

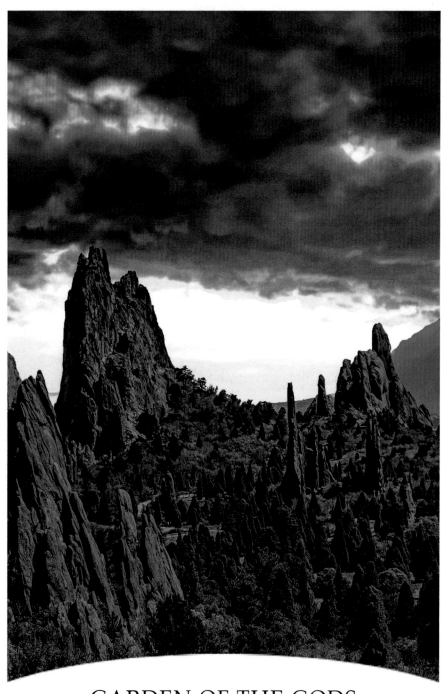

GARDEN OF THE GODS
Colorado, United States

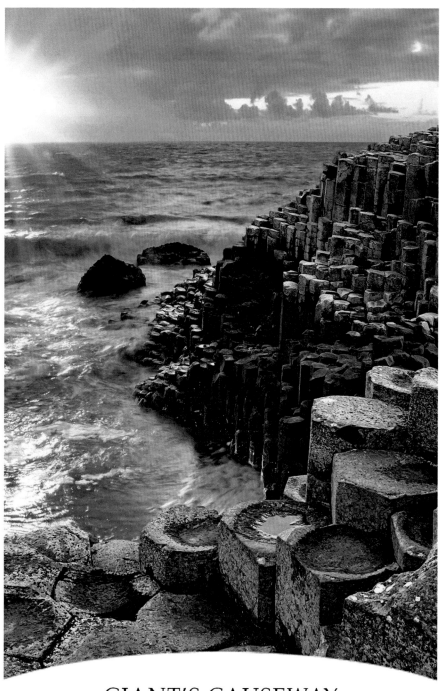

GIANT'S CAUSEWAY
Northern Ireland

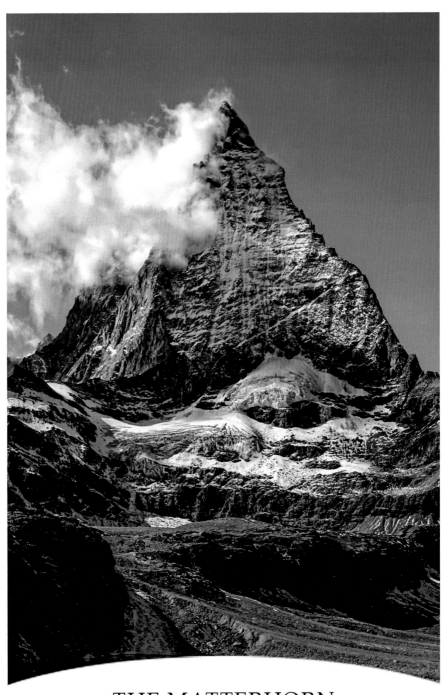

THE MATTERHORN
Switzerland/Italy Border

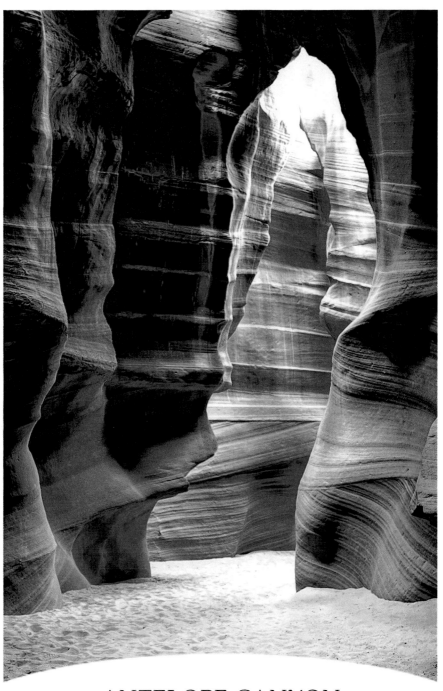

ANTELOPE CANYON
Arizona, United States

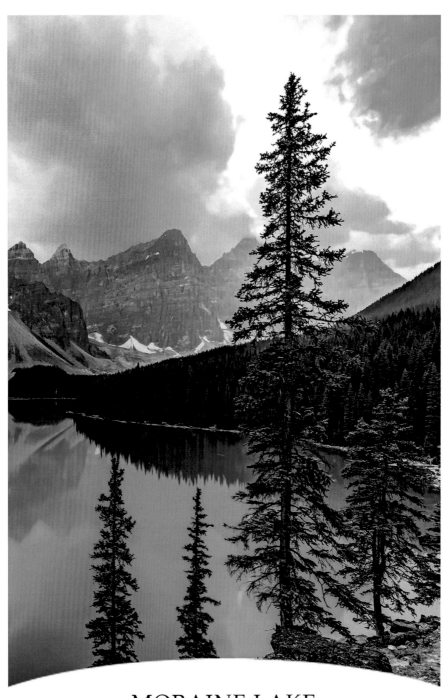

MORAINE LAKE
Alberta, Canada

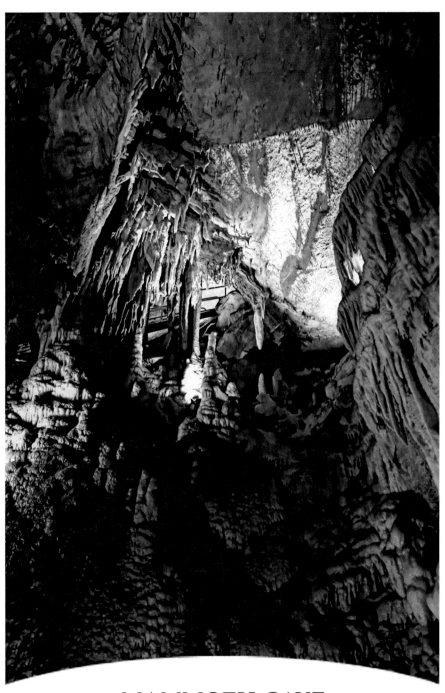

MAMMOTH CAVE
Kentucky, United States

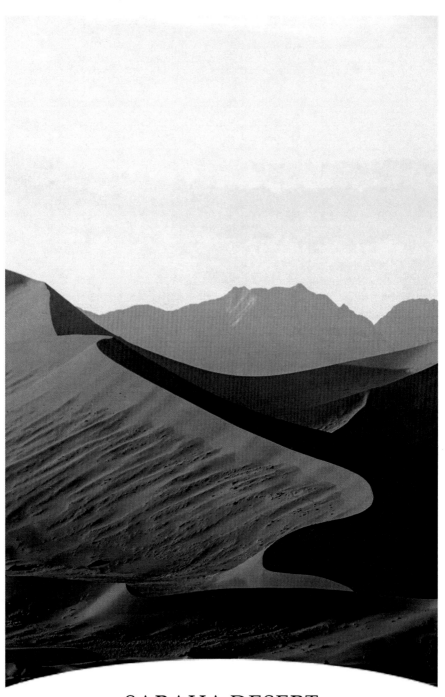

SARAHA DESERT
Namibia, Africa

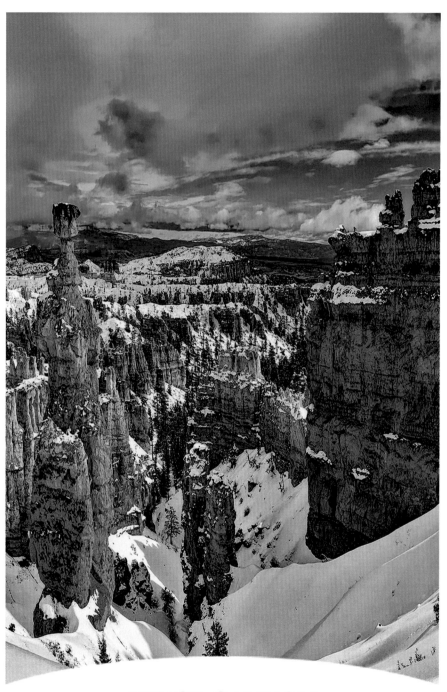

BRYCE CANYON
Utah, United States

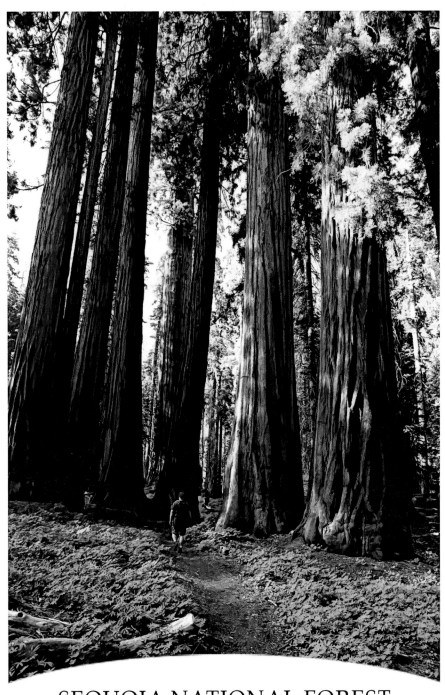

SEQUOIA NATIONAL FOREST
California, United States

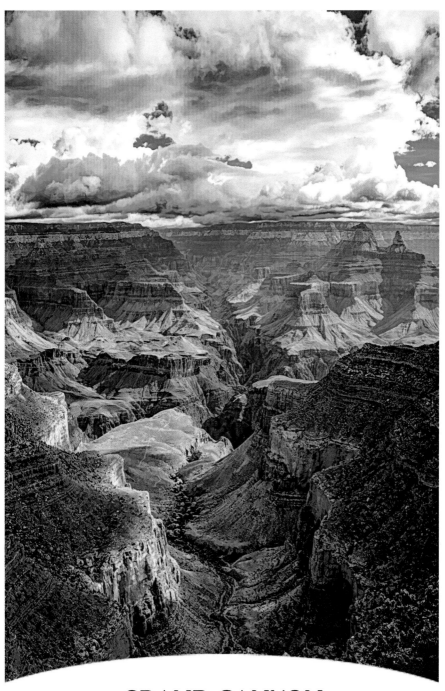

GRAND CANYON
Arizona, United States

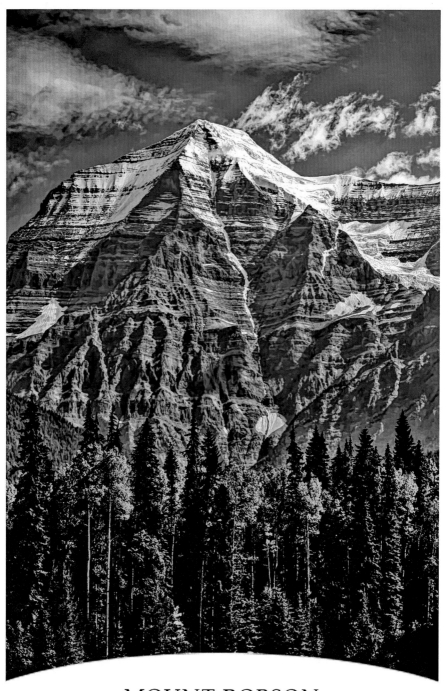

MOUNT ROBSON
Canadian Rocky Mountains

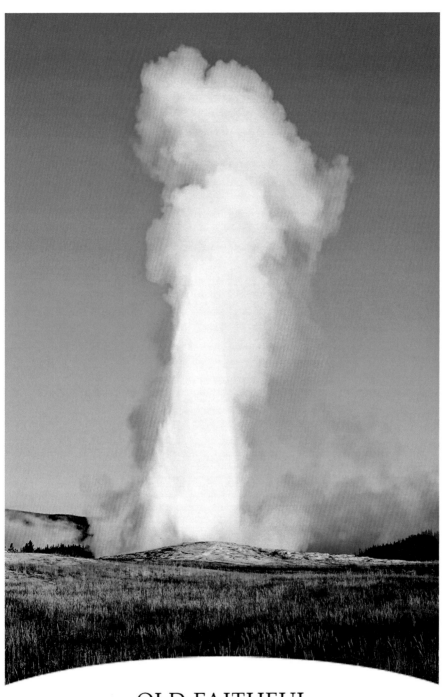

OLD FAITHFUL
Wyoming, United States

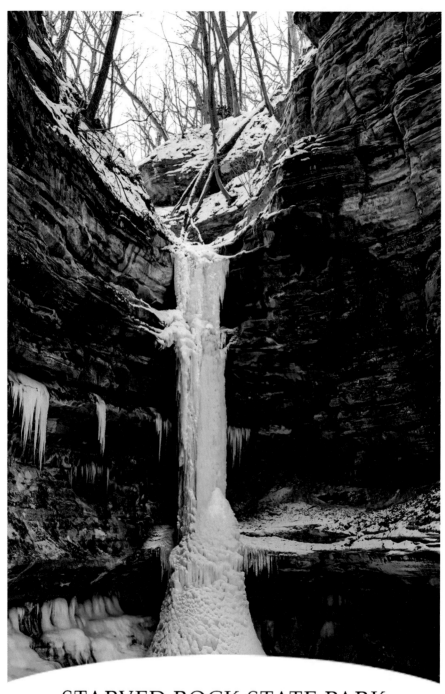

STARVED ROCK STATE PARK
Illinois, United States

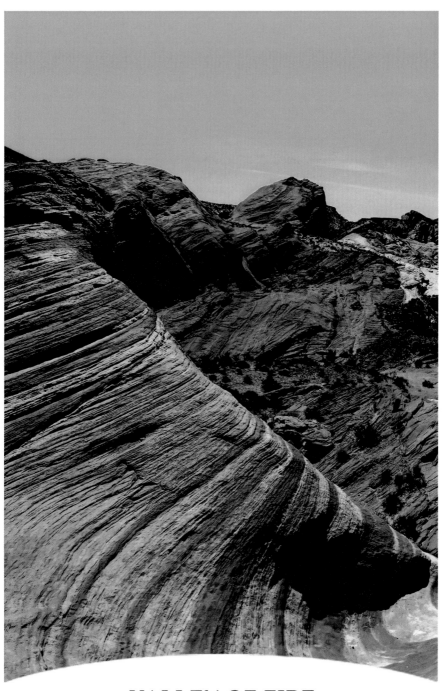

VALLEY OF FIRE
Nevada, United States

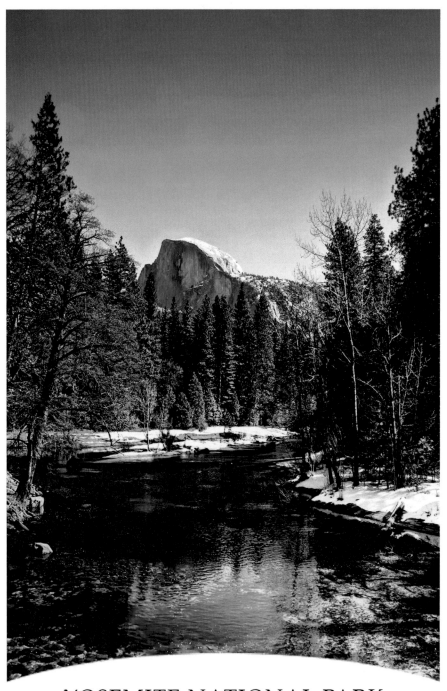

YOSEMITE NATIONAL PARK

California, United States

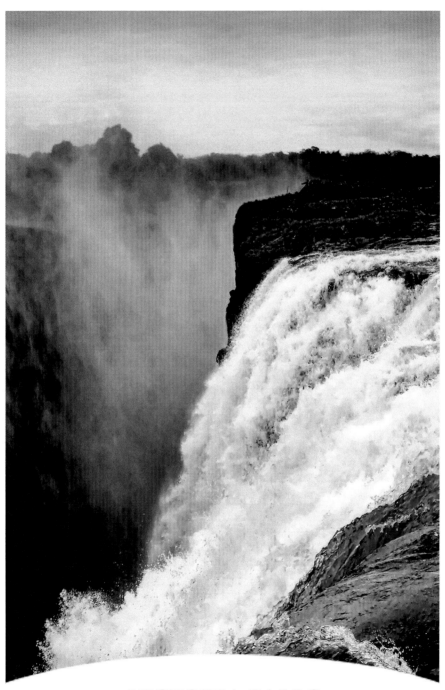

VICTORIA FALLS
Zambezi River, Southern Africa

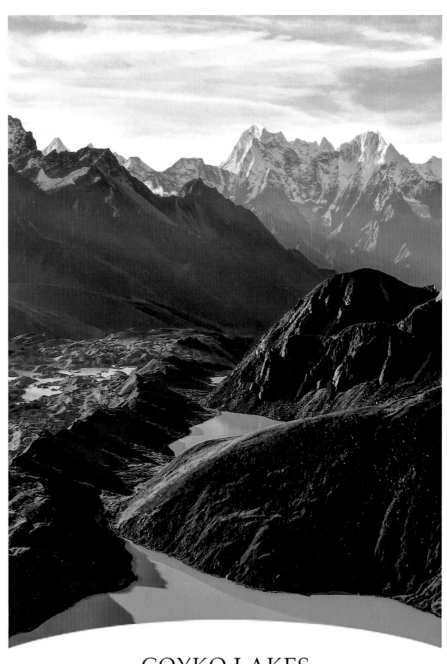

GOYKO LAKES
Nepal

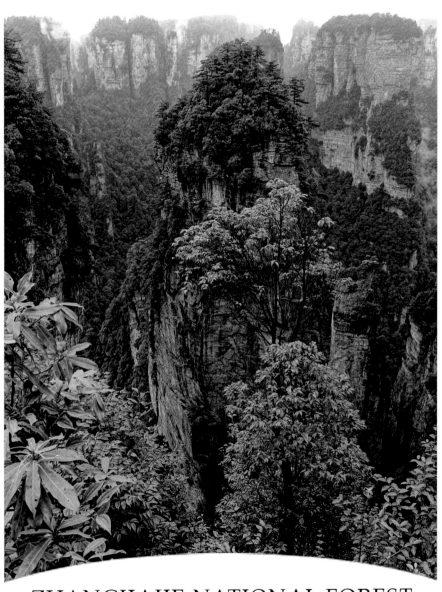

ZHANGJIAJIE NATIONAL FOREST
Zhangjiajie, China

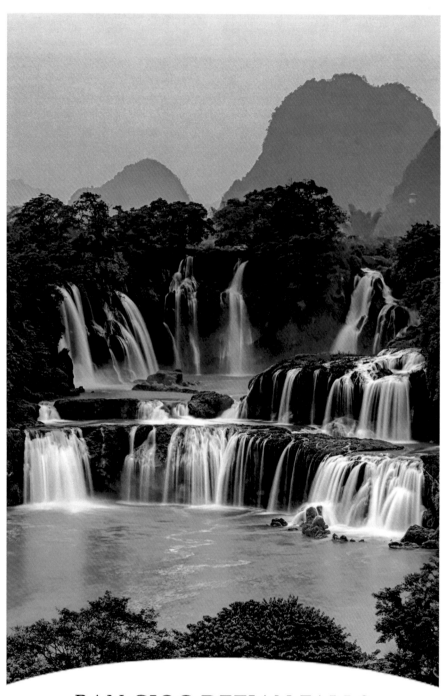

BAN GIOC-DETIAN FALLS
Vietnam / China Border

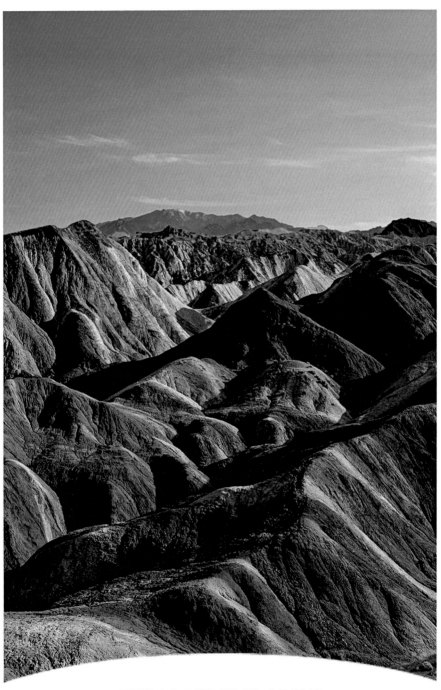

ZHANGYE DANXI
China

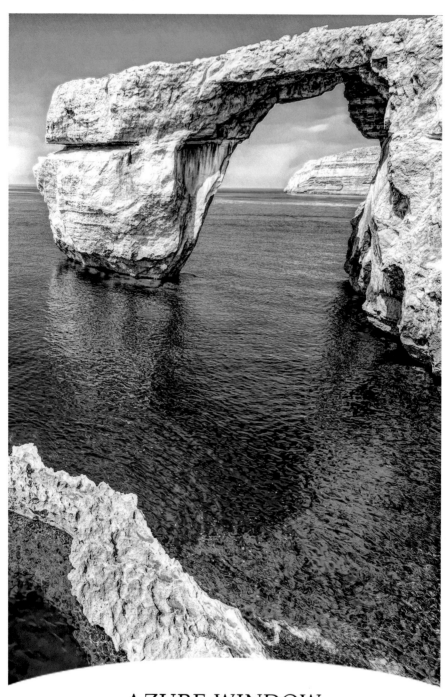

AZURE WINDOW

Malta

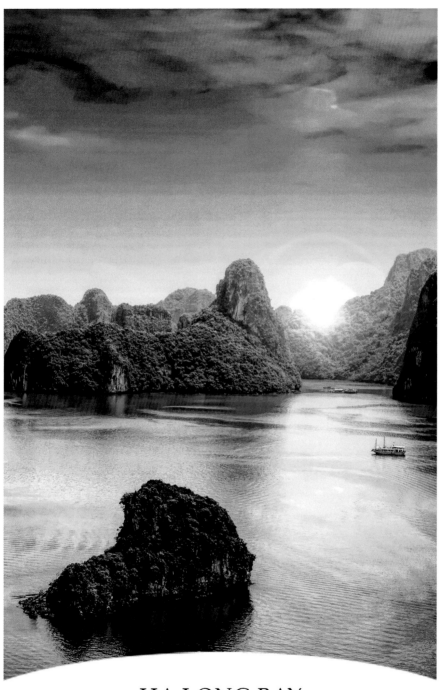

HA LONG BAY
Vietnam

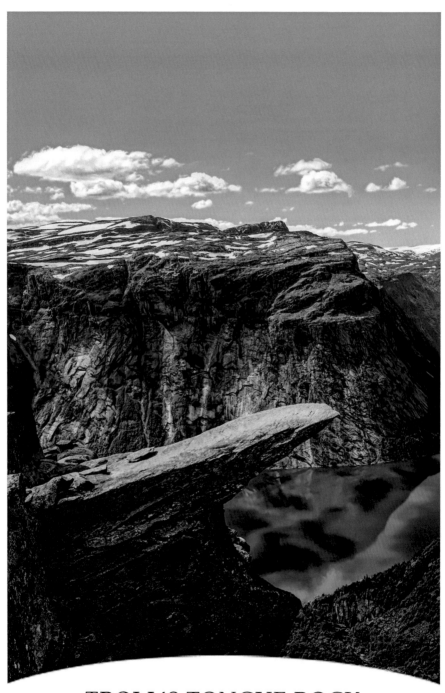

TROLL'S TONGUE ROCK
Norway

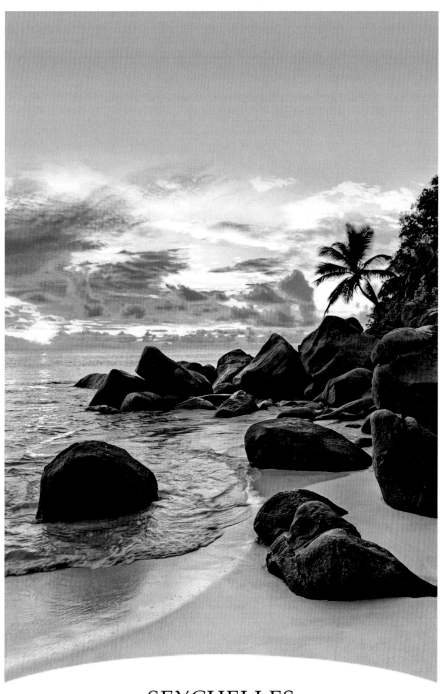

SEYCHELLES
East Africa

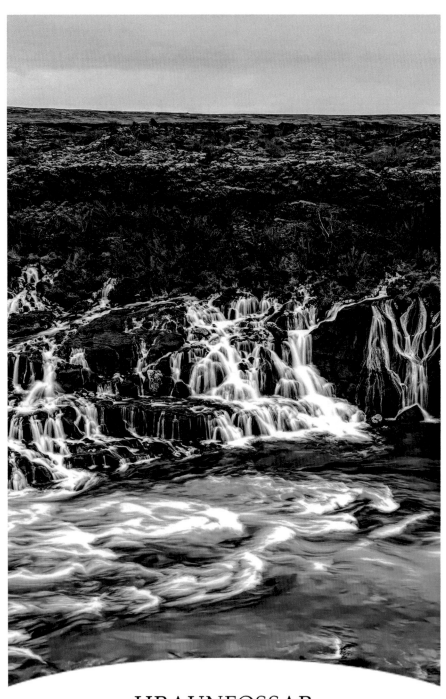

HRAUNFOSSAR
Iceland

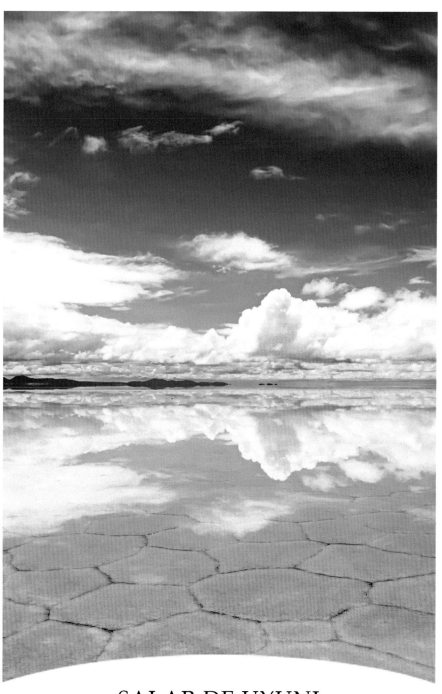

SALAR DE UYUNI
Bolivia

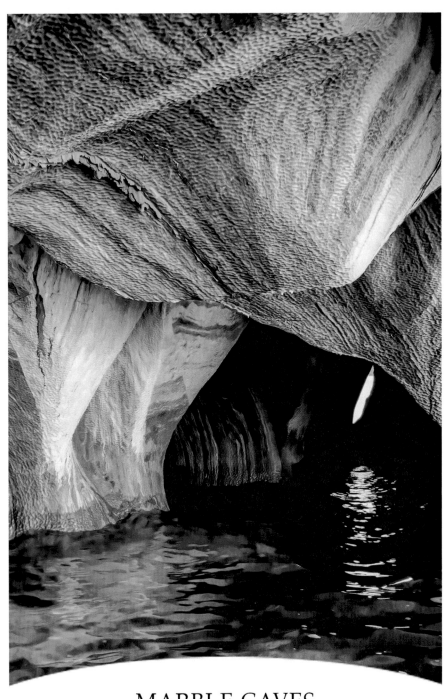

MARBLE CAVES
Southern Chile

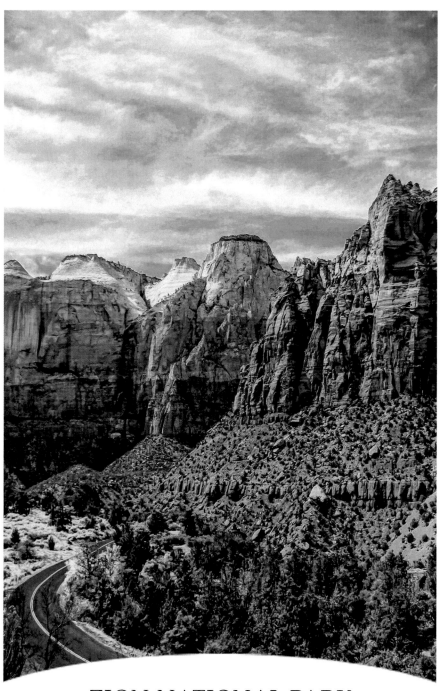

ZION NATIONAL PARK
Utah, United States

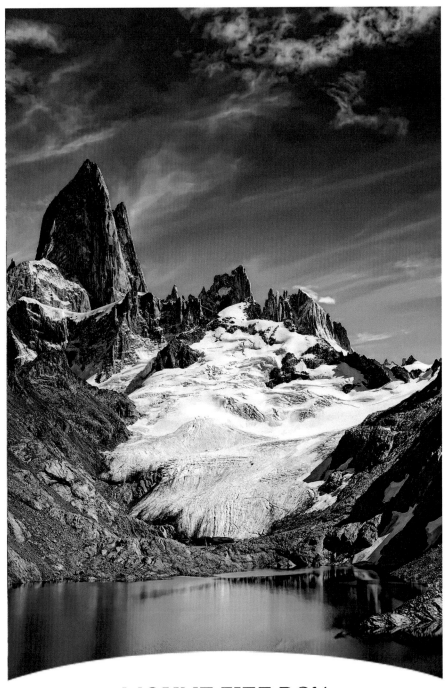

MOUNT FITZ ROY
Patagonia, Argentina

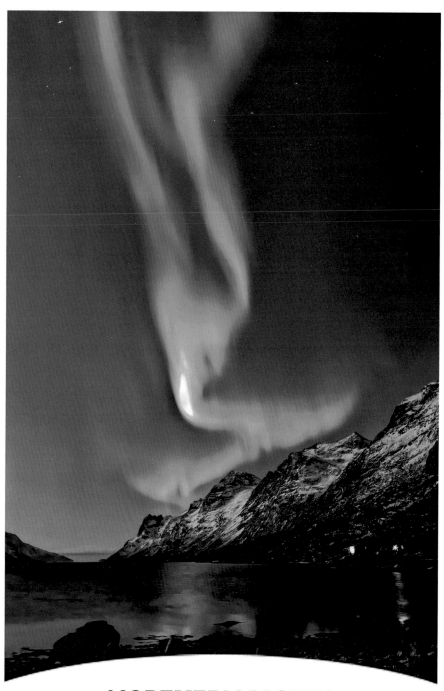

NORTHERN LIGHTS
Norway

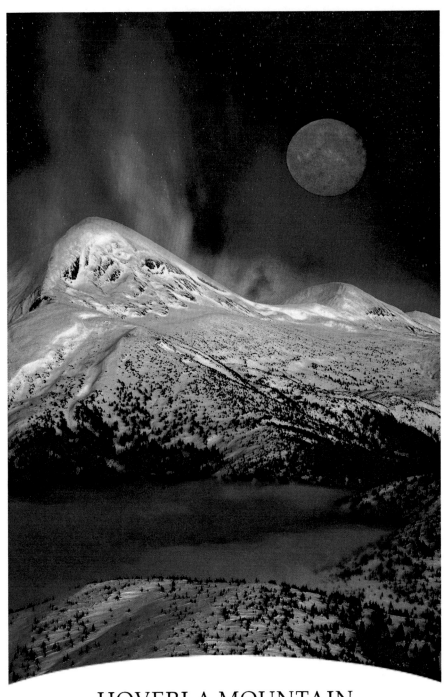

HOVERLA MOUNTAIN
Ukraine

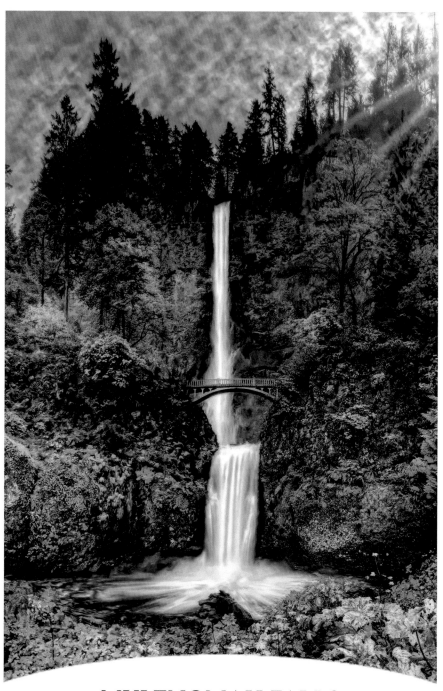

MULTNOMAH FALLS
Oregon, United States